I0411497

HOW TO EAT AND NOT GET FAT

The book to long life and healthy living

P. Karn

Table of Contents

Introduction

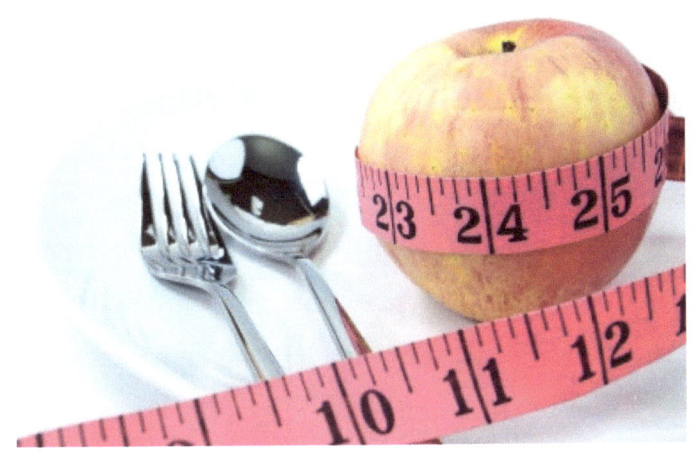

As it is often said, too much of anything is poisonous! Avoid poisoning your health.

You see, most of the time, we bring all sorts of health problems upon ourselves. We adopt unhealthy eating habits and still expect to keep life threatening diseases like obesity at bay. You can exercise all you want but unhealthy eating is exactly that, unhealthy. I am not trying to say that exercising is of no good. I am merely saying that exercising will not compensate for your body's lack of nutrition. Get it?

In order to ensure you live long and enjoy good health throughout your lifetime, you MUST adapt to healthy eating habits.

But must you give up on your treats to be unhealthy? You will find they answer in this e-book.

This e-book seeks to teach you how you can enjoy a long and healthy lifestyle while still enjoying the little pleasures of life. All you need to do is learn how to moderate your intake of these things.

Smart eating is about enjoying your favorite treats and ensuring your body is served with the nutrients it requires to live a long and healthier life.

Chapter 1: What is smart eating all about?

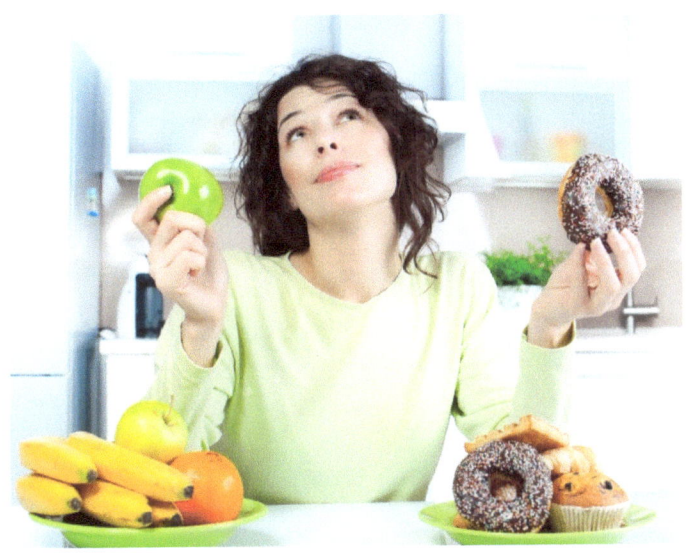

It is not the things you take that kill you; it is about how much you take and how you deal with the excess amounts.

Before you embark on this journey, I will need you to forget everything you have ever heard or read concerning healthy eating, deprivation as well as calories counting. Smart eating is as easy as it is to tuck yourself in at night.

If you have read enough of nutrition and health headlines, you have probably realized that most of these self help books have zero impact on our health. The truth of the matter is that most of us are unhealthy and this is due to bad nutrition choices we often make.

Most of us have tried dietary plans but you only end up fatter than you started off. Take me for example.

A short story of my life

I will let you in on a little story of my life.

Before I was able to discover smart eating as the key to remaining fit and healthy, I tried all sorts of plans. I followed weight loss and nutritional guides that forbid me from eating carbs, the ones that forbid me from eating past 7.00pm and even guides that allowed me to have one meal a day. If I said these plans did not work I would only lie. However, the results were only momentary. The truth is even when you follow these regimens to the letter; life sometimes gets in the way.

Personally, there were a few times I would go into a restaurant and eat more than my regimen allowed. Other times during my normal trips to the self service store I would consume things I was not supposed to consume. The list of the number of times I broke by regimen pact is countless and I am sure you share my sentiments. With time, this leads to frustrations and self hate.

To add to the stress, I would balloon back to my size 16 as soon as I stopped the program. This was quite frustrating since I wanted to lose weight and remain so permanently. After years of trying different weight management and nutrition regimens, I decided I had had enough and I would look for my own ideal way to deal with my weight. It has taken me a while and I have tried various ways to effectively control my weight. Finally, I can comfortably say that I have found the ways to eating without getting fat. I have found my smart eating strategy. And I want to share my findings with you.

The good thing about this strategy is that I do not deprive myself of the little pleasures of life. Today, I am able to enjoy my bar of chocolate and the occasional fried chicken without feeling guilty and fatter.

So, you are probably asking, what is smart eating all about?

Well, to put it simple, smart eating aims teach you how to eat and not get fat. I am here to share my experience with you to ensure you too are able to live free just like I do. I want to prove to you that a little bit of chocolate or junk will not get you fat. It is all about eating management. The problem with us people is that we like taking everything to the extremes. If you do things moderately, you will be able to enjoy it more, for longer.

If you were to look at my before and after pictures, you would find it hard to believe I still get to enjoy my "unhealthy snacks". If you ask me, these snacks will only harm you if you allow them to.

I say, take control of your weight and nutrition, and you will be able to control your whole life.

Want to know how, feel free to flip to the next chapter.

Chapter 2: Taking control of your life

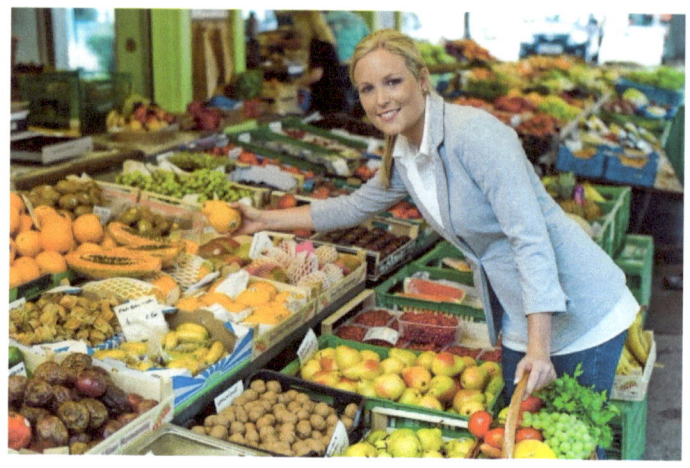

Like it is often said, too much of anything is poison.

The reason health and nutrition is a booming business is because people have developed more interest in nutrition eating. Taking control of your life is all about deciding on what is best for you. It all has to do with discipline. Personally there is no way you will tell me chocolate is bad for my health. I will go ahead and correct you. Chocolate is not bad for my health, too much of chocolate is bad for my health.

I have finally mastered the art of disciplined eating, and you can too. We all have our favorite guilty pleasures. You do not have to give it up, you just have to learn to consume only enough.

Having your cake and eating it too

In my world, it is possible to have your cake and eat it too. Take me for example. I am a heavy eater, especially breakfast. My typical breakfast will comprise of greasy bacon cakes, the chocolate kind (occasionally), two cups of creamy coffee, and a whole bowl of frozen berries, a ripe banana and some form of protein among other things. My breakfast table normally looks like a buffet meal in a restaurant. The best part, I never get fat. Yes! even with all that for breakfast.

You need to realize that, and I did too, eating a heavy breakfast is not equivalent to taking twenty doughnuts. You need to learn how to nutritionally blend your heavy meal, in my case breakfast and other meals. It is also about being sensible about it.

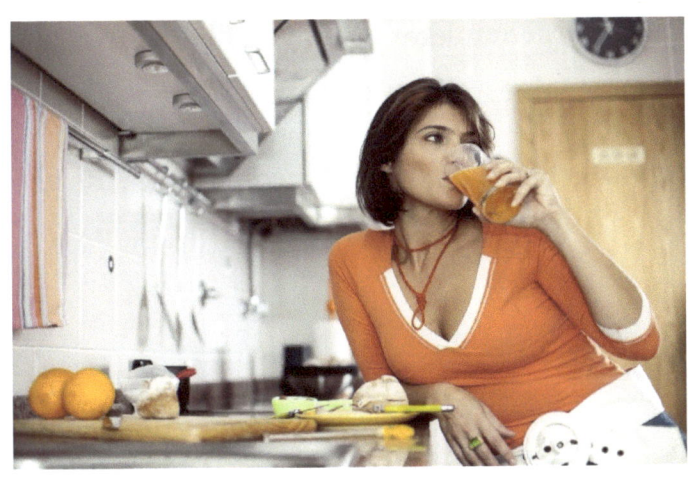

Over lunch time, it will probably have a sandwich, a fruit and a lot of water. This will take me through the afternoon to the evening. When I get home, the first thing I do is take a long walk. This to me is not negotiable. On the days I am not walking, I am running with friends or family. Exercising is a big part of smart eating. It is amazing for your soul, mind and body.

After my walk, I will start on my dinner. For me, dinner mostly comprises of salads, Protein, brown rice and a glass of fine wine. My salads are made of fresh ginger, rosemary, cucumbers, vegetables, bell pepper and cilantro. The dressing is fresh juice made from lime. I avoid using fattening dressings.

This basically completes my day as I look forward to my huge breakfast the next morning.

How do you benefit from this feeding story? Read on.

Your daily meals

Your breakfast

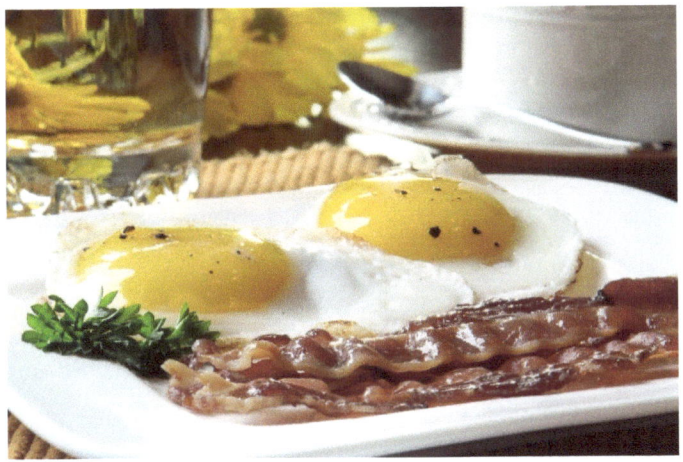

Without a doubt, this is an important meal of the day.
I do not like terming it as the most important meal of
the day since I believe that all meals are important.
While I have a lot to eat at breakfast, I always make it
a priority to make it balanced. A healthy breakfast
should comprise of:

- You favorite snack on occasion.

- Fruit juice.

- A form of protein

- A mug of milk/coffee.

- Brown bread or buns.

This ensures you cover all the nutritional basics. According to me, having a heavy breakfast is essential. This is because it keeps me from eating heavily at lunch and this helps me control my intake of junk. Logically, you are more likely to eat unhealthy snacks if you feel hungry before lunch. I have found this to be the best way to control my junk consumption level.

Your lunch

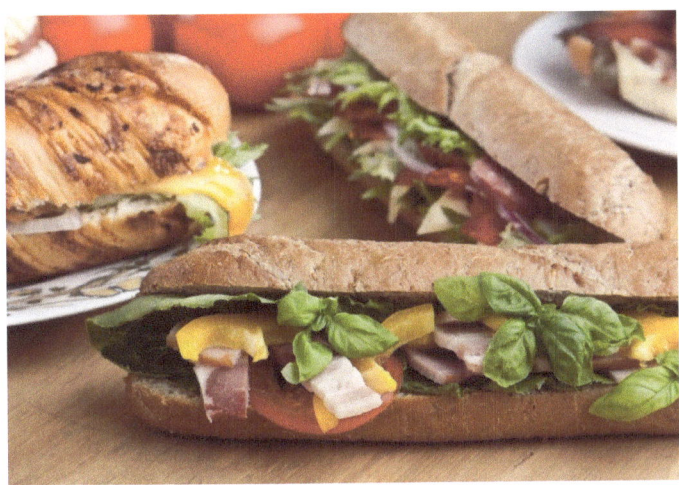

Lunch is also an important meal of the day. Ideally, your lunch should not be that heavy. Just like your breakfast, your lunch needs to be balanced too. An ideal lunch menu should look like:

- A sandwich made from a slice of chicken breast, or a form of protein, vegetables like tomatoes, a few slices of onion, lettuce, and dressing.

- Fresh juice or yogurt.

- Fresh fruits.

- Water.

Ideally, lunch should not be too heavy. You should only have enough to get you through the day. With a breakfast like mine you will probably still feel full by lunch time. Taking a bit at lunch time will again make it easy for you to keep off unhealthy snacks. With this type of lunch, you are probably going to make it through the afternoon and dinner time before you feel hungry.

Your dinner

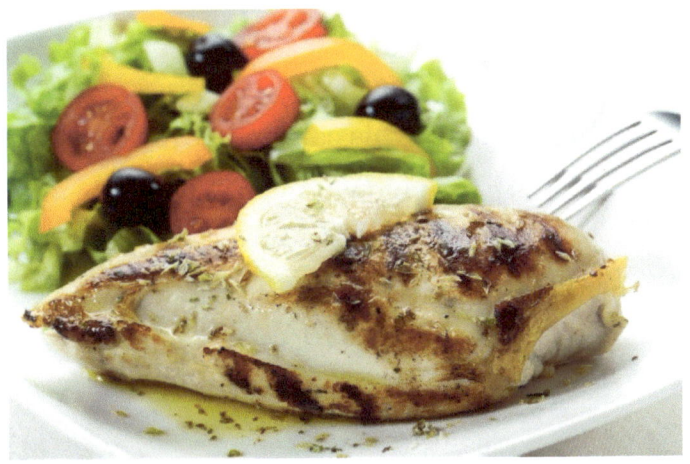

This is yet another meal you are allowed to give it your all. At dinner, you need to eat a bit of everything. Your ideal dinner meal plan should contain the following foods.

- Proteins. This can be chicken, red meat, protein rich grains or fish. I find it better if you try mixing your protein types. If you had chicken at breakfast and lunch, try having fish at dinner. But, if you are a chicken maniac, go ahead and indulge yourself.

- Vegetables. This should make the large part of your dinner. Actually, your dinner plate should be half vegetables.

- Source of fiber. This can be brown bread or rice. It is e to avoid white rice as it unhealthy.

- Vitamins. This can be found in fruits and vegetables. You need to at least have a glass of fresh juice even if you have a plate half filled with veggies.

- A source of carbohydrates.

- Minerals. Avoid diet sodas or any type of sodas. Actually, the best source of minerals is fresh water.

Always ensure your dinner plate is half vegetables. The other half should be divided between proteins and the bread or rice.

I personally believe that planning your meals and following through is the best way to avoid taking unhealthy treats too often. However, this is not about depriving yourself. It is about managing your eating. You can always add a snack between breakfast and lunch or between lunch and dinner. The trick is having them in moderation. I am a chocolate junky but I manage my meals in ways that prevent me from taking the chocolate and other snacks. I have set aside my Wednesdays for my chocolate treat and having it I do.

As for you, what is your little pleasure? Set aside a day or two when you fix the treat in between your meals. This is how I do it. Having my cake and eating it too. The other thing you learn from my meal story is about exercising. That is covered widely in the next chapter.

Chapter 3: About exercising

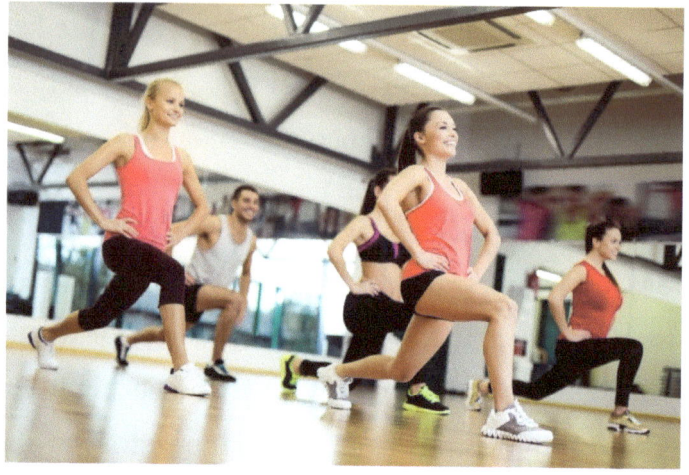

The importance of exercising cannot be underrated. I have found that my heavy breakfast and unhealthy occasional treats without exercising would leave me fat. I understand that there are some people who eat a lot and hardly exercised but still manage to pull a great look.

However, thinking of exercise as a weight loss regimen is a bad misconception. The reason you probably hate exercising is because you have painted a false picture in your head. Before I discovered the secret to weight management, I used to imagine routines and muscle aches. But believe me, my mentality has completely changed.

I finally cracked the code on exercising. It is not about what you do but how you do it. Exercise is fun and helpful. How, you ask?

For me, exercise means doing what I enjoy most, walking. What do you enjoy most?

Choosing what you enjoy doing

You are likely to stick to exercising if you find an activity you enjoy. It is ideal to take some time and think about what you really enjoy doing. This will ensure you look forward to exercising every day.

For most people, thinking of things you like doing is easy. The trick is ensuring it is an activity that makes you move your body. I say this because I realize for some people sitting down and watching TV is their fun time activity. If this is the case with you, then you need to think of something else you like doing. For example just like me you may be a fun of walking, for others it is running while others it is swimming or hiking.

Pairing activities you love to your exercising

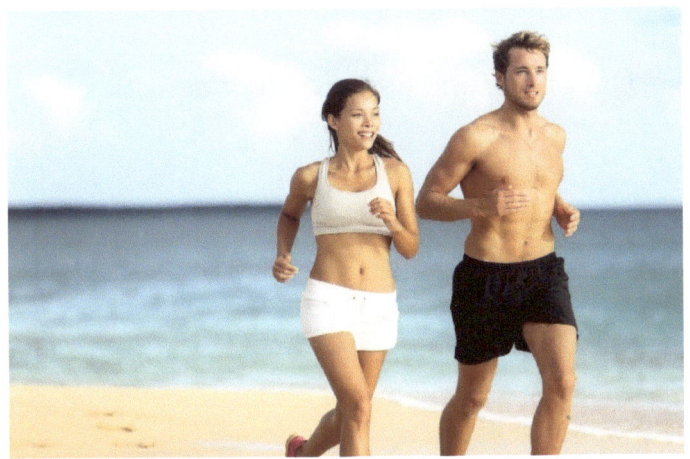

Look around you; you are probably surrounded by fun activities you can exercise through. The trick is finding a fun activity that makes you move your body. When you pair exercising with fun activities, you make it easy and a pleasure.

Some good examples include:

- Taking yoga or dancing classes.

- Dancing to your favorite music.

- Using the treadmill as you watch your favorite program. This is especially helpful to TV addicts.

- Taking jogs with friends and alter on enjoying a movie or coffee treats.

- Gardening and other outdoor activities.

Socializing your workouts

Exercise poses an opportunity for socializing. When you make your workouts social, you are bound to stay motivated and look forward to your sessions every day. Actually, I have found this very ideal. You will find me joining friends for a morning or evening jog.

While socializing, you can cover long distances without feeling the pain. This is because you are talking and catching up. Juicy gossip!

If you are not big on friends, you can join aerobic classes, running clubs or even dance classes. This gives you a platform to socialize as you keep fit.

To spice up your social workouts, you can incorporate competitions. Create a competition and give one another enough time to prepare for it. For instance, my friends and I have a running competition. We set a date for a competition and prepare for it. We make it a complete competition with bets and all. This keeps us motivated and focused. This has really improved the way I look at running. This is coming from a person who considered jogging the best they could do in terms of working their legs.

How do you stay motivated?

One of the hardest tasks human beings are faced with is making behavioral and lifestyle adjustments. It requires patience, effort and time. There are setbacks but you are sure to come out better and stronger is you persevere. At the end of it, you will have benefited physically, mentally and emotionally from exercising.

As a human being, there are times I feel bored and unmotivated to take my daily walks or occasional runs with friends. When this happens, it takes a few things to get my motivation back in check. As much as you like what you do for exercising, it is normal to feel under the weather at times. When this happens, you need to try something new. One of the ways to do this is adding other fun activities to your workout routines. The other way is pursuing your exercises differently.

Setting goals with rewards

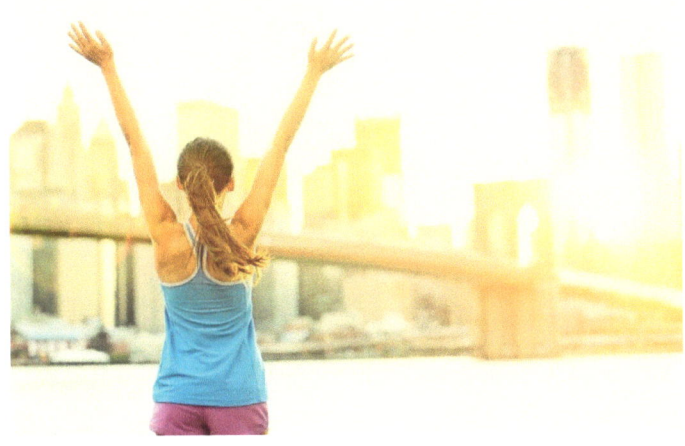

Like I said earlier, I love competitions. If you work out in groups you can have the occasional competitions with rewards. However, setting goals and rewards is a bit different. This is not about competing with your workout partners. It is about setting personal goals and awards.

Goals are important. They act as your driving force towards reaching your goal.

Recently, I wanted to learn a concept regarding my work but I was unmotivated. I decided I would award myself if I learned it within a stipulated time frame. Being a shoeholic, I set my prize at a designer pair that I would die to have. Though it was pricey I decided I would buy it for myself if I managed to learn the concept.

Each time I felt like giving up, I would remember the shoe and just like that I regained my motivation. While I am yet to complete learning the process, I have a few more days to go and I know I'll get the shoe. Fingers crossed!

Equating that to exercising motivation, the concept remains the same. Set a goal to cut a few pounds in a month and work toward attaining it. Also, think of something you really want but have not been able to get and set it as your reward. When you reach this goal, reward yourself and set another goal. I can tell you this, by the time you are done you will have rewarded yourself with everything you wanted.

Keep your exercising going

I understand that times are hard economically and you may not always have the funds to set rewards. I don't always set rewards. Even with rewards, it sometimes gets old and you see it as normal. There are other ideas I use, and hopefully you can use too to keep on exercising.

Ensure consistency - remaining consistent is a challenge to most of us. The best way to make it consistent is to exercise at the same time every day. For me, I have to take my walks before dinner and after work. With time, you body adapts to your timing and you will find it very hard to go a day without exercising.

Recording progress – it is important to keep a recording journal for your exercises. In a few months, you can go through your journal and see the changes you have made. I am warning you, this can be seriously motivating.

Maintaining the fun - every time you think of your exercise session, see it as your alone time or time with friends. Make it interesting; listen to music, change locations and chat with your friends. Above everything, ensure you workouts never become boring.

Spreading the word – talk to people you trust about your latest exercising and your goals. This will keep you motivated because you know there is someone waiting to celebrate with you when you reach your goals.

These tips are sure you keep you going even in times you want to give up. They have been very helpful to me.

You may be wondering why I have emphasized much on exercising. The reason is simple; there is a rich connection between exercising and your ability to enjoy your 'unhealthy treats'. This we discuss in the next chapter. Read on!

Chapter 4: Relationship between exercising and smart eating

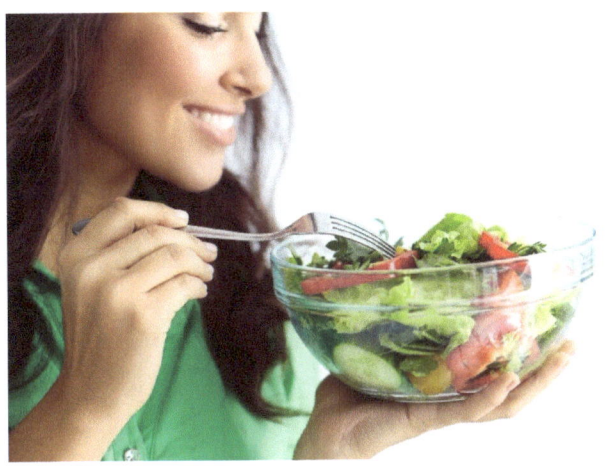

There are numerous benefits you get from regular exercising. To you and me, one of these benefits is the ability to enjoy our treats. Again, the reason I emphasized so much on exercising is because it is the aspect that makes it possible for me to take a heavy breakfast and not get fat. It is the aspect that will allow you to enjoy your unhealthy pleasures and still maintain your ideal body weight.

Basically, exercising burns calories. I don't know about you by my little pleasures come packed with those. Remember above we said that you are allowed to enjoy treats once or twice a week. This ensures that your daily exercising burns the calories that you acquire from these snacks. The intensity of your workout will dictate how many calories you burn per workout. This is why I emphasize on exercises that make you sweat.

Why smart eating without exercising will make you fat

Before I learned of the advantages involved in exercising and why it is ideal to incorporate it in my eating habits, I thought, no, I had convinced myself that I do not need exercise. I imagined that learning to control my eating was all I needed to cut the extra pounds. But I was proved wrong a few months later.

If you are like me; sticking to healthy meals with the occasional snacks plus the hope of not getting fat, I am here to ask you to wake up from your illusion. You can cut or replace your snacks for healthy alternatives all you want but it is a complete waste of time if you do not exercise.

Apart from my own personal experience that I am sharing, scientists have also proven this to be true. Dieting does not cause weight loss, at least not substantially. Smart eating goes hand in hand with exercising. There is really no other way around it.

With most people, eating and not exercising actually makes them fat. This is because exercising burns fat and calories leaving you slimmer with time. Lack of exercising means that fewer calories are being burnt to provide energy for your daily activities. The rest of the calories and fat are stored in the body meaning you get fat. It is really as simple as that.

With your occasional 'unhealthy snack', you really don't want that fat stored in your body.

Personally, I had tried the smart eating strategy for three or four months before I realized I seriously needed exercising. Before this, I had tried to look through the internet for motivation that I could actually enjoy my snacks, healthy eating and weight loss without exercising. The internet can be quite convincing since I got results like who needs exercising with healthy eating and remain fit without exercising and all manner of results. These results kept me going for a while before I decided to cease lying to myself. After four months, I had only lost 1 ½ kilograms. This had to be my wakeup call.

With time I started looking into different ways to exercise and this looked promising and so I kept at it until I finally figured it out. This is how I have been able to compile this e-book for you dear reader.

Clearly, there is need for each one of us to take control of our eating habits. This is the only way you and I can eat and not get fat. If it has worked for me, it will work for you. You only have to start now.

Conclusion

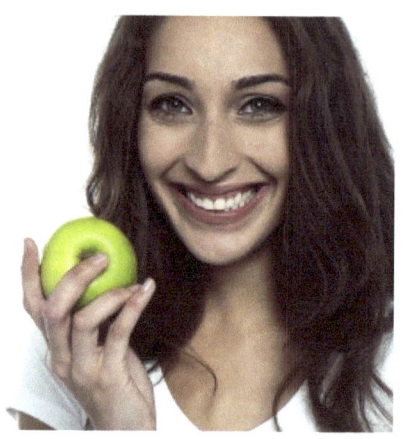

You have been with me from the first chapter and by now you have understood the need for you to take control of your eating. This e-book proves beyond reasonable doubt that it is possible for you to eat and not get fat. You can enjoy your guilty pleasures without worrying about getting fat.

Remember it is not about not enjoying your favorite 'unhealthy snacks' but it is all about learning to control how you enjoy them.

Just like I said in the beginning, it is not the things you take that kill you, it is about how much you take and how you deal with the excess amounts.

A little bit of anything never hurt anybody!

www.ingramcontent.com/pod-product-compliance
Lightning Source LLC
Chambersburg PA
CBHW040746010626
45792CB00027B/584